12 STEPS TO A PAIN-FREE BACK

By

Ray C. Mulry, Ph.D.
Clinical Psychologist and Executive Director
American Network Services
Tustin, California

Arthur H. White, M.D.
Orthopedic Surgeon and Medical Director
St. Mary's Spine Center
St. Mary's Hospital and Medical Center
San Francisco, California.

Eugenia A. Klein
Editorial Coordinator

A SIGNET BOOK

NEW AMERICAN LIBRARY

TIMES MIRROR

PUBLISHER'S NOTE
The ideas, procedures, and suggestions
contained in this book are not intended as a
substitute for consulting with your physician.
All matters regarding your health require
medical supervision.

 SIGNET TRADEMARK REG. U.S. PAT. OFF. AND FOREIGN COUNTRIES
REGISTERED TRADEMARK—MARCA REGISTRADA
HECHO EN SECAUCUS, NEW JERSEY

SIGNET, SIGNET CLASSIC, MENTOR, PLUME, MERIDIAN and NAL
BOOKS are published by The New American Library, Inc.,
1633 Broadway, New York, New York 10019

First Printing, November, 1983

1 2 3 4 5 6 7 8 9

PRINTED IN THE UNITED STATES OF AMERICA

Contents

Introduction

Low back pain can be prevented, treated, and rehabilitated with the programs of exercise and relaxation in this book. Following these programs step by step may free you from the certainty that old pains will keep coming back—and turn the pain you may be enduring right now into a distant memory.

Do not rush yourself. Your back will return to health as you expand your learning over time. So be prepared to follow an orderly sequence of ideas and exercises. Be sure to read the entire book thoroughly.

12 Steps to a Pain-Free Back has four parts:
1. Know Your Back
2. Manage Your Tension
3. Strengthen and Stretch Your Body
4. 12 Steps to a Pain-Free Back

The parts all work together as a "total person" approach to low back problems. This approach follows accepted medical guidelines. You can practice all the treatments safely in your own home. Of course, as with any health program, you should check with your physician before you begin. Once you have your physician's go-ahead, all that's required is your desire and determination.

After you have learned how to protect your back, you may never have to endure back pain again.

1 Know Your Back

Learn how to move about safely. Spare yourself pain and begin to restore your back to fitness by keeping these important principles of everyday movement firmly in mind: balance and protective body mechanics, strengthening, and stretching, and rest.

Consider these principles for a moment—one at a time.

Balance

If you are swayback, hunchback, or overweight, or if you spend long periods of time in awkward working positions, chances are your spine is not in balance. Being off balance can cause excessive wear on a portion of your spine. The result is almost always back pain.

So it's important to concentrate on even your simplest daily movements because your back is constantly at work—and at risk. Pushing, pulling, reaching, bending, lifting, twisting, sitting, lying down, standing, and walking all require proper balance. Make a habit of thinking about the effect your movements are having on your back. Make balance a daily watchword. Remind yourself to balance your spine frequently throughout your day. Your efforts will begin to pay off right away.

Take a close look at the following illustrations to see how to balance yourself during daily living. Practice the *right* way in front of the mirror. The general rule for good balance of the spine is to keep your back straight, pull in your stomach, tuck your buttocks under, and bend your knees.

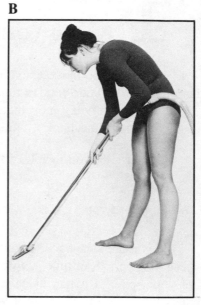

Pushing and/or pulling.
A. Right: back straight, stomach in, buttocks under, and knees bent.
B. Wrong: back bent and knees locked.

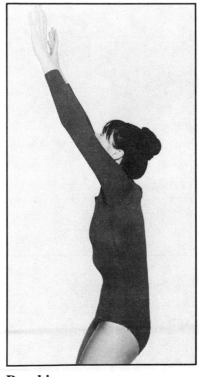 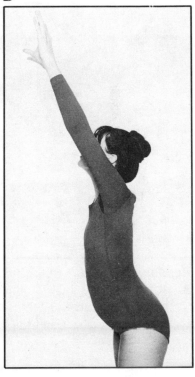

Reaching.
A. Right: back straight, stomach in, and buttocks under (knees bent).
B. Wrong: swayback.

A

B

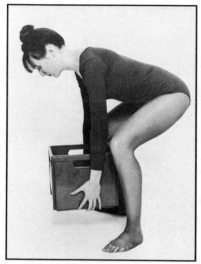 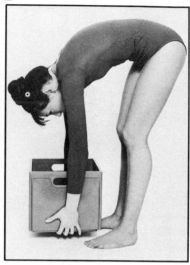

Bending or lifting.

A. Right: back straight, stomach in, buttocks under, and knees bent.

B. Wrong: back bent and knees straight.

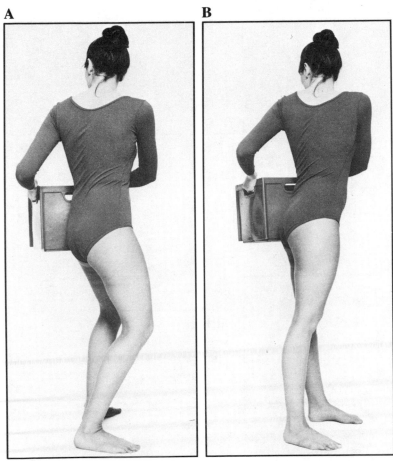

Twisting.
A. Right: turn shoulders, hips, and feet together.
B. Wrong: feet planted and shoulders not in line with hips and feet.

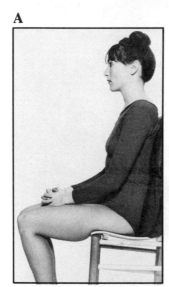

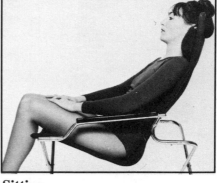

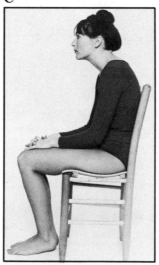

Sitting.
A and **B.** Right: low back
supported and straight.
C. Wrong: back bent.

A

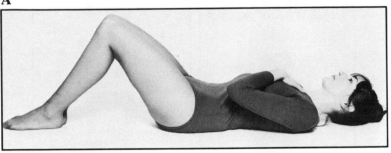

B

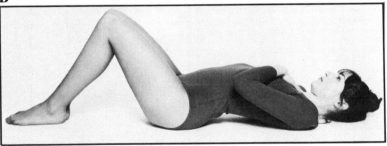

Lying.
A. Right: back straight and knees bent.
B. Wrong: back swayed.

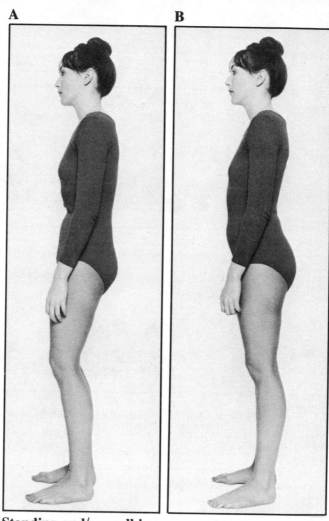

Standing and/or walking.

A. Right: back straight, stomach in, buttocks under, and knees bent.

B. Wrong: swayback and knees straight.

Protective Body Mechanics

Certain body positions safeguard you against injury when you're performing physical tasks. These efficient, advantageous positions are known as *protective body mechanics*. You can put them into action immediately by learning the following postures: the *Pelvic Tilt* and the *Straight-Back Bend.*

The Pelvic Tilt: The Pelvic Tilt is an excellent example of protective body mechanics. In general, it corrects poor posture. But beyond that, it is your spine's basic protection during physical activity.

Four maneuvers are involved:
- Back straight
- Stomach tightened
- Buttocks tucked under
- Knees bent

Back straight means keep your spine in an upright or vertical position when performing a task. Don't "round" the back.

Stomach tightened means use your stomach muscles to support your spine from the front of your body when performing a task. By tightening your stomach muscles, you press your stomach against the spine, giving it extra support and preventing it from bending. Tightening the stomach is the real key to success with your back. It is the focus of all your self-protective exercises.

Buttocks tucked under means bring your lower spine into a straight line position.

Knees bent means allow your legs (thighs) to serve as shock absorbers when you are lifting, moving, carrying, or accepting heavy loads. If you put your thighs to work, you lessen the physical strain on your spine.

To get maximum benefit from the Pelvic Tilt:

- Do not let your shoulders sag too far forward.
- Do not throw your shoulders back into a military position. (This causes a swayback.)
- Tighten your stomach muscles—pull them in.
- Hold your head in a straight line with your spine. Do not allow your head to protrude or fall forward.
- Do the Pelvic Tilt frequently. It's a simple position that will bring predictable comfort to your spine.

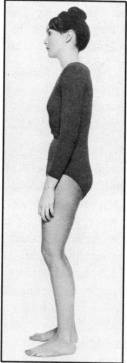

Pelvic Tilt: back straight, stomach in, buttocks tucked under, and knees bent.

The Straight-Back Bend: Although protective body mechanics usually implies maintaining your spine in an upright or vertical position, this is not always possible. There are situations, such as removing packages from the trunk of a car, that require another kind of protective maneuver. This particular maneuver is called the *Straight-Back Bend*. Between the Pelvic Tilt and the Straight-Back Bend, you should be able to perform most physical tasks without unusual wear or strain on your lower back. Keep your back straight.

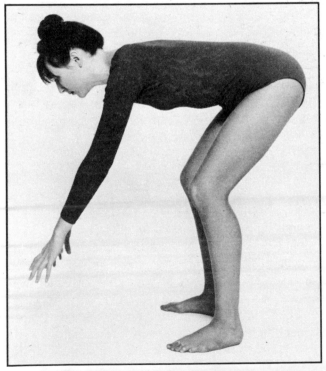

Straight-Back Bend: back straight, stomach tightened, and knees bent.

Rest

Rest does not necessarily mean sleep. Rest also refers to times when you want to relax your muscles. At those times your spine needs special support. Learn the rest positions that will help:

- When sitting, use a reclining or contour chair or a straight chair with pillows supporting your lower back.
- When standing, lean against a wall in the Pelvic Tilt position.
- When lying down, lie on your side in a contour position or on your back with a pillow under your knees. Put a pillow under your waist to keep the spine from sagging when you are resting on your side.

Be Kind to Your Back!

- Realign your body many times throughout the day.
- If you sit at a desk all day or work in a bent over position, change your position frequently, stand up, stretch, and move around. The stretches in your Daily Maintenance Program are very useful during these everyday work situations. Your body gets tight/tense during the day. Proper and frequent stretching is essential to good care of your back.

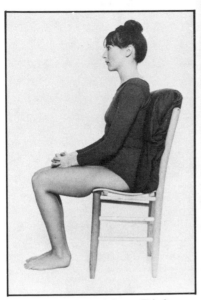

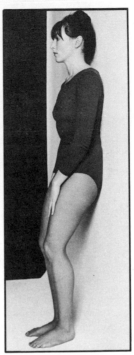

Sitting rest position. Right
way to sit with low back
supported and straight.

Standing rest position.

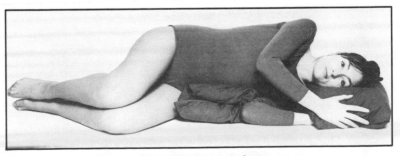

Lying rest position with pillow at waist.

2 Manage Your Tension

When you are stressed, angry, or generally frustrated, your muscles can become tight or tense. We want to show you how to take control of your stress so you'll learn:

- How to identify sources of stress in your life
- How to reduce negative stress
- How to relax your muscles

When you are having trouble with your back, it is important to remember you are not just muscles, bones, and nerves. You are also a feeling human being. Understanding your emotions is as important to the care of your back as anything else.

When you are happy, joyful, relaxed, and full of buoyant feelings, you move with flexibility and ease. On the other hand, when you feel angry, depressed, tense, and burdened with frustrations and personal concerns, you tighten up, restrict yourself, and struggle with the world around you.

Stress and Tension in Everyday Life

Noise, financial pressures, problems with children, marital problems, time pressures, medical bills, and trouble with your employer are a few potential stressors. Anything that makes your heart work beyond its normal pace, makes you perspire, or causes your muscles to tighten may be considered a stressor.

Stress, however, can be either positive or negative.

Positive stress is any influence that disrupts bodily balance,

PERSONAL CONCERNS

A Program

DATE _____

SEX _____ AGE _____ HEIGHT _____ WEIGHT _____

MARITAL STATUS _____

	DAY 1	DAY 2	DAY 3	DAY 4	DAY 5	DAY 6	DAY 7	TOTAL	DAY 1	DAY 2
Need More Recreation										
Noise At Home										
Noise At Work										
Sleeping Problems										
Chest Pain										
Problems With Children										
Weight Problem										
Need to be More Assertive										
Recent Death in Family										
High Blood Pressure										
Conflicts With Relatives										
Poor Eating Habits										
Short Temper										
Freeway Traffic										
Cigarette Smoking										
Feel Guilty										
Back Pain										
Alcohol (self)										
Alcohol (other)										
Jealousy										
Pill Consumption										
Boredom										
Tension										
Worry Too Much										
Medical Bills										
Need Employment										
Divorce										
Separation										
Dislike Job										
Continued Physical Pain										
Job Security										
Unexpressed Anger										
Headaches										
Trouble Making Decisions										
Conflicts With Neighbors										
Marital Problems										
Financial Difficulties										
Desire More Social Life										
Need to Relax										
Trouble With Employer										
Need Physical Exercise										
Need Friends										
Nervousness										
Sex Difficulties										
More Time for Myself										
Deadlines on Job										
Depression										
Can't Say No										
Ulcers										
Loneliness										
General Unhappiness										
More Self-discipline										
TOTAL										

INVENTORY
of Self-Study

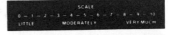

SCALE

0 — 1 — 2 — 3 — 4 — 5 — 6 — 7 — 8 — 9 — 10

LITTLE   MODERATELY   VERY MUCH

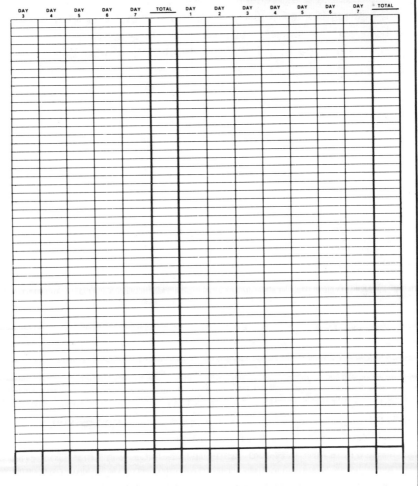

DAY 3	DAY 4	DAY 5	DAY 6	DAY 7	TOTAL	DAY 1	DAY 2	DAY 3	DAY 4	DAY 5	DAY 6	DAY 7	TOTAL

23

yet still leads to a strengthening of physical functioning. If you go jogging, your heart rate will typically increase, you will perspire, and your muscles will tighten. If you exercise intelligently, you will make your body stronger and healthier.

Negative stress is any influence that disrupts bodily balance and leads to a weakening of physical functioning. For example, if you jog beyond your limits, you may damage or weaken your body and, of course, your general health condition.

What you want in your daily life is a comfortable amount of positive stress and no negative stress. And before you can reduce negative stress, you have to identify its sources.

Your Personal Concerns Inventory

To identify sources of negative stress, rate yourself daily on the Personal Concerns Inventory on pages 25–30. See which stressors are causing problems for you on a given day, and which persist from one day to the next. These persistent stressors are the critical ones, especially if they are causing you a high degree of concern.

Use the scale to rate each listed item from zero to ten, zero meaning the issue causes you little concern and ten meaning it concerns you very much. We would consider any rating over seven as indicating a high degree of concern.

Your daily rating for each item should be made at the end of the day and should reflect your experience on that day. You may be unsure which rating to start with on a specific item. That does not matter because you are free to change your mind the next day and to increase or decrease your rating as you feel it accurately represents your true concern.

There are fifty-two items listed in the Personal Concerns Inventory. When you fill out the inventory for the first time, read the following brief descriptions carefully, then insert your rating into the chart. If you are unsure whether or not you are concerned with a specific item, just ask yourself if the issue causes you tension and or worry. If it does not, you may assign it a rating of zero.

1. Need More Recreation _____
Are you concerned about your need for fun or playtime?

2. Noise at Home _____
Does the noise level at home bother you? Have you noticed this before as a potential source of tension? Does the noise from traffic, airplanes, television, voices, dogs barking, or other such sounds bother you?

3. Noise at Work _____
Is your work situation quiet and pleasant, or is noise (typewriters, voices, traffic, hammering) a factor in your daily personal balance?

4. Sleeping Problems _____
Did you sleep well last night? Did you use sleeping aids? Were you rested when you woke up?

5. Chest Pain _____
Have you noticed any pain in your chest today? If so, are you concerned about it?

6. Problems With Children _____
Of course, you care about your children, but have you been *concerned* or *worried* about them *today?*

7. Weight Problem _____
Are you the right weight for your good health? Did your weight bother or concern you today?

8. Need To Be More Assertive _____
Did you let opportunity slip by because you were too passive to stand up for yourself? If so, does this concern you?

9. Recent Death in Family _____

It is possible you have recently experienced a death in the family, and it is also possible this does not concern you. Be honest with yourself and rate the item appropriately.

10. High Blood Pressure _____

Do you know your blood pressure? If so, does it concern you?

11. Conflicts With Relatives _____

Have relatives (other than your spouse or children) been a source of tension for you today?

12. Poor Eating Habits _____

Do you eat regularly and maintain a healthy diet?

13. Short Temper _____

Did you find yourself particularly on edge today? Did you lose your temper?

14. Traffic _____

Did the noise, congestion, speed, and general activity on the road bother you today?

15. Cigarette Smoking _____

Are you a smoker? Does this concern you? This does not refer to someone else's smoking because there is very little you can do about that.

16. Feel Guilty _____

Did you experience guilt feelings today? Does this concern you?

17. Back Pain _____

Did you experience back pain today? If so, how important is this to you, and did you do anything about it?

18. Alcohol (self) _____

This refers to your own drinking habits and how well you

manage yourself when you are drinking. Even if you did not have a drink today, you may still be concerned about this issue in terms of your personal habits and general tendencies.

19. Alcohol (other) ———
Did someone else's drinking bother you today?

20. Jealousy ———
Did you feel jealous today? If so, does this concern you?

21. Pill Consumption ———
Are you taking pills more than necessary or in a way contrary to medical advice? This does not refer to vitamin pills or any other pill that is prescribed by a physician for a specific medical condition such as diabetes or thyroid problems.

22. Boredom ———
Were you bored today? Was your day rather pointless?

23. Tension ———
Was this a tense day for you? Did your tensions get out of hand?

24. Worry Too Much ———
Did you feel worried today? Is this becoming a concern of yours?

25. Bills ———
Are you concerned about accumulating bills?

26. Need Employment ———
Are you concerned about finding a job?

27. Divorce ———
Did you have thoughts about an ongoing or pending divorce today? Is this a concern of yours?

28. Separation ———
Did you have thoughts about an ongoing or pending separation today? Is this a concern of yours?

29. Dislike Job _____
Did your work situation annoy you today? Do you feel satisfied with what you are doing in your job?

30. Continued Physical Pain _____
Has a continuing pain such as headache, backache, or chest pain been on your mind today?

31. Job Security _____
Do you feel secure in your job?

32. Unexpressed Anger _____
Are you concerned about angry feelings that you keep inside?

33. Headaches _____
Did you have a headache today? Are you concerned about this?

34. Trouble Making Decisions _____
Do you go back and forth and find it difficult to take decisive action?

35. Conflicts With Neighbors _____
Are the neighbors getting on your nerves?

36. Marital Problems _____
Are you and your spouse getting along? If not, how much does this concern you? If you are not married, you may relate this item to an important ongoing interpersonal relationship.

37. Financial Difficulties _____
Did money pressures bother you today?

38. Desire More Social Life _____
Do you feel the need for more leisure time with others?

39. Need To Relax _____
Are you attending to your need for relaxation? Is this something you postpone?

40. Trouble With Employer _____
Are your working relationships satisfactory?

41. Need Physical Exercise _____
Are you aware of your needs for adequate physical exercise?

42. Need Friends _____
Are you concerned about feelings of friendship? Did this issue surface for you today?

43. Nervousness _____
Were your nerves on edge today?

44. Sex Difficulties _____
Are you concerned about the adequacy of your sex life?

45. More Time for Myself _____
Do you feel the need to be alone and pursue your own interests?

46. Deadline on Job _____
Did deadlines and time pressures get to you at work?

47. Depression _____
Did you feel down and depressed today?

48. Can't Say No _____
Did you find yourself doing things you did not want to do because you were unable to say no to someone?

49. Ulcers _____
Were you concerned about ulcers today?

50. Loneliness _____
Did you feel lonely and in need of people in your life today?

51. General Unhappiness _____
When you take all things into consideration, do you feel your life is generally in balance?

52. More Self-discipline _____

Very little changes for the better unless you exert yourself in a growth-oriented manner. Are you doing what you need to do to bring your life into balance?

Now that you have made fifty-two self-assessments, add them up to determine your *total personal concerns score*. Each day, as you total your ratings, you can see whether your overall level is increasing, decreasing, or staying the same. The goal, of course, is to lower your score as much as possible.

All items rated 7, 8, 9, or 10 are your primary concerns. Secondary concerns have ratings of 3, 4, 5, and 6. Ratings of 1 and 2 are not significant enough to require immediate attention.

Primary concerns are your most significant trouble spots and indicate where you can make the most constructive changes in your daily routine. You may want to discuss them with your physician and a consultant who specializes in your area of concern.

Could a few adjustments in your daily life help your back? Think about it! Your mind can do wonderful things.

When you learn to manage stress and tension, your body responds by lowering your heart rate, decreasing your blood pressure, and stabilizing your flow of adrenaline, thus allowing your muscles to relax. Learning to handle stress and tension improves your physical *and* emotional health.

Make a conscious decision to manage your stress and tension. Self-control is part of proper back care. Make relaxation a goal, and follow up on it every day.

For some of us, of course, relaxing is easier said than done. Maybe you need to develop better relaxation skills to free yourself from the many stresses you encounter daily.

If so, then Relaxation Therapy is a good way to begin the process. Relaxation Therapy is a simple way to reduce muscle tightness and emotional tension.

Here's what to do:

Relaxation Therapy

1. Find a quiet, comfortable place where you can relax your body completely. You may choose a bed, the floor, a comfortable chair, or any other place that is convenient.
2. Lie on your back. Be sure your back is in a straight-line position. Place two pillows under your knees to flatten your lower back. A small pillow or a rolled towel under your neck will give you the support you need for your head and neck.
3. Close your eyes. Breathe according to your own natural rhythm, letting each deep breath fill you with peaceful, soothing relaxation. Now slowly take a deep breath to the count of four and expand your stomach diaphragm, thus allowing more space for your lungs as they fill with air. Now exhale slowly through your mouth to the count of eight. Relax. Repeat this procedure four more times

Position for Relaxation Therapy.

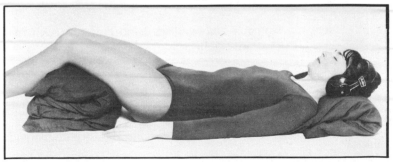

and notice how you are already enjoying the deepening relaxation.

4. Let all the tensions drain from your body, particularly in muscle areas causing you discomfort or stress. Concentrate on the process.

5. Now, slowly, start counting backward from five to zero. With each descending number you will feel more relaxed. To focus your thoughts, try saying these words as you count:

Five . . . five . . . five . . . I feel relaxed.

Four . . . four . . . four . . . I feel tranquil and at peace.

Three . . . three . . . three . . . With each deep breath I feel more and more relaxed.

Two . . . two . . . two . . . My body feels limp and relaxed.

One . . . one . . . one . . . I am entering a deeper and deeper state of relaxation and am feeling quiet and sleepy.

6. Feel the tension draining from your body. Notice how the muscles throughout your body are relaxed. Once again, follow this script to focus your thoughts:

My head and neck muscles are becoming loose, limp, and relaxed.

The muscles throughout my back are loose and relaxed.

Now my stomach and waist are loosening up. All the muscles in my midsection are relaxed.

The area around my hips feels loose and relaxed. The area in front and back of my hips is totally loose and relaxed.

My relaxed feelings are progressing into my thighs and legs and down into my feet.

Muscle tightness is disappearing and I feel limp, loose, and at ease.

7. Now imagine a pleasant scene where you feel content and relaxed. Allow your mind to find its own place of peace. Allow your mind to wander to any enjoyable image or thought until you feel like returning to a more active state.
8. When you feel like opening your eyes, take a deep breath and slowly open them. Savor your renewed energy. Enjoy that relaxed sense of well-being.
9. Proceed with your activities of daily living with a renewed sense of personal balance and a feeling of "centeredness."

Questions and Answers

Should I try to do anything during Relaxation Therapy?

No, just have a pleasant time. Let yourself go, and you will relax regardless of whether or not you are concentrating on the words and procedures of Relaxation Therapy. Relaxation Therapy is, in many respects, a *process of letting go*. Do not interfere with this process if you can help it.

Do I need a teacher to do Relaxation Therapy?

No, this text is sufficient. Allow your own experience to be your guide, and learn to trust yourself.

I often feel guilty when I take time out to relax. What can I do about this?

Remember, you are a more rewarding person to others when

you are relaxed, balanced, and free of discomfort. You have a *right to a restful time alone*.

Does Relaxation Therapy require any self-discipline?

Yes. It may seem strange to you, but you will have to take time out from your daily schedule to do Relaxation Therapy. Self-regulation does require self-discipline.

How long should a Relaxation Therapy session last?

Fifteen to twenty minutes is long enough, but you may want to continue the deep state of rest. This will be determined by how much your body is in need of additional rest and relaxation.

Does it make any difference if I do Relaxation Therapy daily?

Yes. Relaxation Therapy is a process that helps you help yourself. Daily relaxation is essential to your overall care of yourself. If you are more tense than usual or are in the early stages of caring for your back, you may do Relaxation Therapy two or even three times a day. Let your needs for relaxation be your guide, and don't wait until you are overly tense.

Is Relaxation Therapy the most important part of the total Tension Management® program?

No, Tension Management® is the integration of stressor identification skills with relaxation skills so you will cope more effectively with daily stresses and tensions.

Perhaps the most important aspect of Tension Management is that you do what needs to be done so you establish effective and lasting solutions to your personal concerns.

How often can or should I do Relaxation Therapy?

You can do Relaxation Therapy as often as you like. It cannot harm you.

Should I do Relaxation Therapy before I go to sleep at night?

You have undoubtedly heard the advertisements, "Relax and go to sleep." If you want to rid yourself of sleeping pills, Relaxation Therapy will be of considerable benefit to you.

Can I relax too deeply and not wake up on my own?

No, your body has its own regulatory system. You will not relax too much, and you will wake up when you are ready. Incidentally, many people *fall asleep* during Relaxation Therapy. This is a good result. Sleep is a form of deep relaxation and something most people with back pain need.

Is Relaxation Therapy the same as biofeedback?

No, but biofeedback is also a process through which you can learn to relax. You may also use biofeedback as another form of self-help. One of the advantages of Relaxation Therapy is that you can do it at any time and also in the privacy of your home.

Can I also meditate if I want to?

Yes. Anything that helps you to relax and feel good about yourself is useful to you.

How long does it take to respond to Relaxation Therapy?

Most people respond during their first session. Almost everyone will relax fully in two or three sessions.

3 Strengthen and Stretch Your Body

You have decided to take control of your pain. You are ready to start feeling better—and keep on feeling better.

You have learned how to keep your spine in balance. How to relax. How to protect your back from injury. How to control stress and tension.

Now you are ready to round out your total back care program with our *12 steps to a pain-free back*—12 exercises that will strengthen and stretch your body.

Why does your back need exercise?

All joints are protected by surrounding muscles, and your spinal column is no exception. The lower back is protected by four major muscle groups. These muscle groups include:

- *Gluteal* or *buttock* muscles
- *Quadriceps* or *thigh* muscles
- *Abdominal* or *stomach* muscles
- *Paraspinal* muscles, or muscles that parallel the *spinal* column

In order to maintain a healthy back, you need strengthening exercises for the first three muscle groups.

Your paraspinal muscles are probably well developed already. Frequently these muscles are also tight. When they become longer and more flexible, you have greater flexibility of body movement in general. So you also need stretching exercises for your paraspinal muscles.

The 12 exercises we have given you are keyed to programs that match your symptoms. No matter which program you choose, you achieve the greatest benefit if you follow these guidelines:

- Be sure you can do any given exercise painlessly before you move on to the next. Be patient with yourself.
- Complete your Personal Concerns Inventory and practice Relaxation Therapy on a daily basis.
- Remember to use all the techniques of balance, protective body mechanics, and relaxation that you learned in the first chapter of this book as you go through your daily activities.
- Contact your physician when you have new pain or pain that does not decrease with the help of exercise. Many of the conditions that cause new back pain are potentially serious and require the aid of a physician. There are many things a physician can do to help you resolve such pain safely and rapidly while you practice our program.

Identify Your Program

Choose the program that matches your symptoms, then follow the exercise treatment prescribed. We explain how to do these exercises in Chapter 4.

New Pain Program I

Symptoms:
Back pain with spasm or crookedness
Little or no leg pain
No numbness, tingling, or weakness
Treatment:
1. Do Exercise 12, the McKenzie Press Up, also known as

the cobra exercise in yoga. Repeat every hour for as long as necessary.

2. Do this exercise as painlessly as possible. At first your low back discomfort and tightness will probably intensify a little, but the pain area should decrease in size and intensity and eventually disappear. If pain increases, spreads, or fails to disappear, begin bed rest (see New Pain Program II, steps 1–2) and notify your physician.
3. Do not sit or bend your spine forward during this treatment or for several days afterward. You may recline in a reclining chair or rocking chair with a small pillow or support behind your lower back to make your back arch backward.
4. Once you have been pain-free for one week, begin Exercises 1–4 for stretching and range of motion.

New Pain Program II

Symptoms:

    Any new low back pain

    Shooting leg pain, numbness, tingling, weakness

Treatment:

    Your pain will probably go away in a few weeks. However, once you have had back pain, you will most likely have a recurrence. Therefore the following program is of great importance to you:

1. Lie down in your most comfortable position—a contour position on your side (see page 19), or on your back, with pillows under your knees (see page 31). Stay in these positions as much of the time as possible. It sometimes takes several hours in the proper position for the pain to subside.

2. Change positions slowly. Tighten your stomach muscles before moving. Roll on your side and push yourself to an upright position as painlessly as possible. Sit as little as possible. Stand in the position of greatest comfort. Because of your pain you may not be able to stand straight. Give in to the position your body is telling you is least painful. Walk only for short distances, to go to the bathroom or get something to eat. Return to the lying position that is most comfortable. Stay as free of pain as possible.

3. After you are able to function without pain medication, you can resume your daily activities. You should sit, stand, and walk only in the correct positions. Increase your activities painlessly without the use of pain medication.

4. Begin your recovery program with Exercises 1, 2, 3, and 4. Do these painlessly. If they cause pain, stop doing them and seek the attention of your physician. You should be able to move around the house in a pain-controlled manner and take short walks and limited drives in a car.

5. When you can painlessly perform Exercises 1 to 4 as prescribed, add Exercises 5, 6, 7, and 8 to your routine. If they cause any pain, stop immediately. The following day there may be some muscle soreness, but there should not be any increase in your back pain or spread of your back pain in any direction. You should now be ready to go back to office work, do housework, participate in some recreational activities such as swimming and bicycling, resume sexual activity, and travel.

6. When you have been pain-free for three months, you may advance from this program to the No Pain Program.

Old Pain Program

Symptoms:
> Mainly moderate low back pain
> Recurrence of minor symptoms

Treatment:

Your back pain is not likely to disappear spontaneously. You will have to make some major changes in what you do for your body on a daily basis.

1. Do Exercises 1 to 4 until you have achieved twice the normal recommended levels for Exercises 1 and 2 and until you can maintain a Wall Slide Hold (Exercise 3) for 1 minute and a Partial Sit-up (Exercise 4) for 1 minute.

2. Proceed to Exercises 5 to 8. Your pain should decrease by following the preceding recommendations. If the pain does not decrease, seek the attention of your physician.

3. When you have been pain-free in normal daily activities for several months, you may add Exercises 9 to 12, as long as you are able to do them painlessly. There is a limit to what your back will allow you to do but you should be able to swim, bicycle, play tennis, and play golf. Renewed pain will tell you when you may be doing these activities improperly. Speak with your physician.

No Pain Program

Symptoms:
None
Possible vague low back discomfort or concern for physical fitness and prevention of back pain
Treatment:
1. You are pain-free and want to stay fit. You can probably do Exercises 1 to 12 completely. Do them slowly. Do not overexert yourself. Immediately stop doing any exercises that cause pain.
2. Maximum success in this exercise routine will require ongoing Tension Management®. Continue practicing Relaxation Therapy and complete your Personal Concerns Inventory on a daily basis.

Daily Maintenance Program

Proper back care requires a continuing strengthening and stretching exercise program. Do these 12 exercises in the following order, once in the morning and once in the evening, only after completing your specific program.
1. Wall Slide Hold—3 minutes
2. Partial Sit-up—3 minutes
3. Moving Squat—30 seconds
4. The Standing Hamstring Stretch—30 seconds

5. The Full-Body Groin Stretch—30 seconds
6. Repeat the Moving Squat—increase to 45 seconds
7. Repeat the Standing Hamstring Stretch—increase to 45 seconds
8. Repeat the Full-Body Groin Stretch—increase to 45 seconds
9. Repeat the Moving Squat—increase to 60 seconds
10. Repeat the Standing Hamstring Stretch—increase to 60 seconds
11. Repeat the Full-Body Groin Stretch—increase to 60 seconds
12. The McKenzie Press Up—10 repetitions held for 5 seconds each.

The Moving Squat and the Standing Hamstring Stretch can be done at any time during the day to counteract muscle tightness.

Remain relaxed. Relaxation leads to stretching, and stretching leads to relaxation. Never push or rush yourself while stretching. The quality of the stretch is far more important than the number of stretches.

4 12 Steps to a Pain-Free Back

These exercises are keyed to your individual program (see Chapter 3). Follow your program carefully and *do not do any exercise that causes pain*.

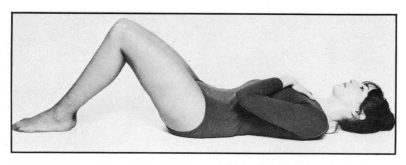

EXERCISE 1: Pelvic Tilt on Your Back

1. Lie on your back with your knees bent.
2. Flatten the small of your back by tightening the stomach muscles and tilting your pelvis.
3. Tighten your buttocks.
4. Hold this position for 10 seconds. Repeat 10 times.
5. The Pelvic Tilt will be performed as the first step in each exercise.

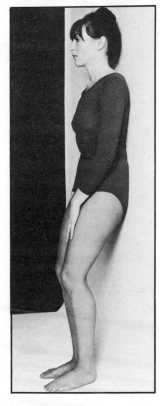

EXERCISE 2: Pelvic Tilt Against the Wall

1. Stand with the small of your back *flat* against the wall.
2. Place your heels 12 inches from the wall.
3. Pull in your stomach.
4. Tighten your buttocks.
5. Bend your knees.
6. Hold this position for 10 seconds. Repeat 10 times.

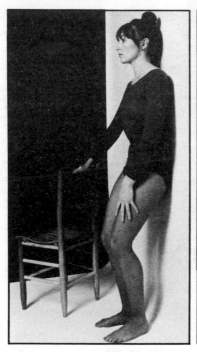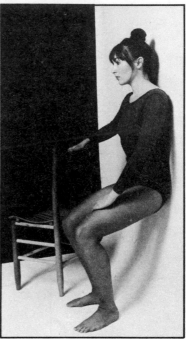

EXERCISE 3: Wall Slide Hold

1. Stand with the small of your back flat against the wall.
2. Place your heels 12 to 18 inches from the wall.
3. Pull in your stomach.
4. Bend your knees and slide 6 to 8 inches down the wall.
5. Hold this position for 10 seconds.
6. Return to the standing position by sliding back up the wall. Repeat 10 times. Relax and walk around between repetitions.
7. Progressively increase your distance down the wall until your thighs are at a 90-degree angle to the wall.
8. The minimum holding time goal at a 90-degree angle is 1 minute.
9. Eventually increase holding time in the 90-degree angle position to 3 minutes.

Note: Do not do Exercise 3
if you have any problem
with your knees.

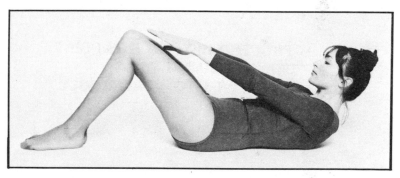

EXERCISE 4: Partial Sit-up

1. Lie on your back with your knees bent and in the Pelvic Tilt.
2. Reach for the top of your knees and lift your shoulder blades off the floor.
3. Hold for a count of 10.
4. Return to the start position and relax.
5. Gradually increase your holding time capacity to 3 minutes.
6. If you have any neck pain be sure to tuck your chin in toward your chest.

Note: If this exercise aggravates neck pain, STOP.

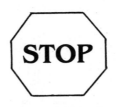

**DO NOT PROCEED BEYOND THIS POINT
UNLESS YOU ARE ABLE
TO DO EXERCISES 1 TO 4 PAINLESSLY.**

The *stretching* exercises on the following pages have been carefully selected to help you find a systematic method for achieving greater flexibility.

Learning how to stretch properly so you do not injure muscle tissue is essential to this stretching program. Stretch up to the point of pain but not beyond that point.

Relaxation is the first step in stretching. Concentrate on the feeling of relaxation and allow that feeling to spread throughout the muscle group you are about to stretch. *You must learn that straining, bouncing, pulling, and other similar movements have no place in your stretching activities.* Your breathing should be slow and easy and a flowing part of your stretch. In other words, you are engaged in a natural activity that will lead to the relaxed letting go of muscle tissue.

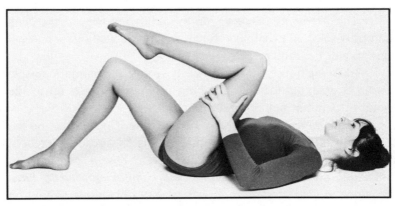

EXERCISE 5: Knee to Chest

1. Lie on your back with your knees bent in the Pelvic Tilt position.
2. Place both hands behind the thigh and pull gently and slowly toward the chest, exhaling as the knee comes up.
3. Relax and hold for a count of five.
4. Release and inhale as the leg returns to the start position.
5. Repeat with the other leg.
6. Do five repetitions with each leg.

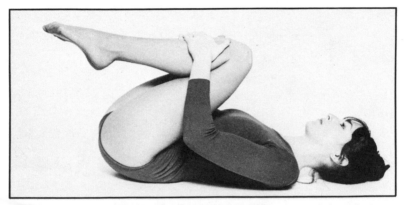

EXERCISE 6: Both Knees to Chest

1. Lie on your back with your knees bent in the Pelvic Tilt position.
2. Place both hands in front of your knees and bring both knees to the chest, exhaling as the knees approach the chest.
3. Relax and hold for a count of five.
4. Release and inhale as your legs return to the start position.
5. Repeat five times.

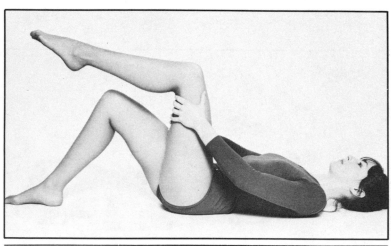

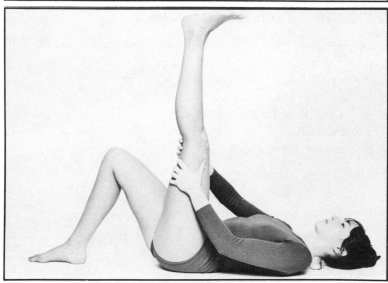

EXERCISE 7: The Hamstring Stretch

1. Lie on your back with your knees bent in the Pelvic Tilt position.
2. Bring one knee *toward your chest*, exhaling as the knee comes up. Reach forward with both hands and hold behind the knee.
3. Straighten your leg upward.
4. Hold for a count of five. Bend the knee and return to the start position.
5. Repeat with the other leg.
6. Do five repetitions with each leg.

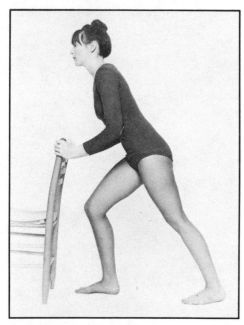

EXERCISE 8: The Heel Cord Stretch

1. At arm's length, face the wall, a desk, or other sturdy object.
2. Place one foot 12 inches behind the other with both heels planted firmly on the floor.
3. Lean into the wall or object.
4. Keep your back straight.
5. Stretch the heel cord and hamstring of the rear leg by leaning forward over the front foot.
6. Hold for 5 seconds.
7. Alternate with the other leg.
8. Do each leg five times.

IF YOU CAN PERFORM ALL
STRENGTHENING AND STRETCHING EXERCISES
CORRECTLY AND PAINLESSLY,
ADD EXERCISES 9 AND 10.

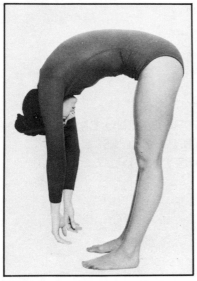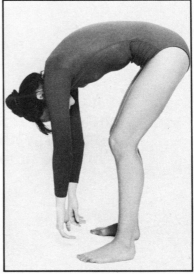

EXERCISE 9: The Standing Hamstring Stretch

1. Stand up straight with your feet a shoulder's width apart.
2. *Slowly* bend forward at the waist.
3. Let your head, neck, and arms hang freely.
4. Relax into the stretch for 30 seconds.
5. Do not bounce when doing this stretch.
6. *Bend your knees* and return to the standing position.
7. Repeat this exercise and continue the stretch for 45 seconds.
8. Repeat this exercise and continue the stretch for 60 seconds.
9. Be sure to let your neck and head hang loose.

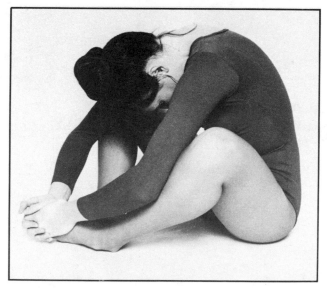

EXERCISE 10: The Full-Body Groin Stretch

1. Sit on the floor and place the soles of your feet together.
2. Grasp your toes and gently pull your heels toward the groin.
3. Place your elbows in front of your shins. Hang your head loosely.
4. Relax into the stretch for 30 seconds.
5. Repeat for a 45-second stretch.
6. Repeat for a 60-second stretch.

IF YOU ARE ABLE TO PERFORM
ALL PREVIOUS EXERCISES PAINLESSLY,
ADD EXERCISES 11 and 12.

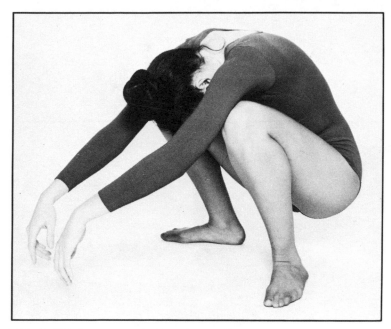

EXERCISE 11: The Moving Squat

1. Stand with your feet flat on the floor, 6 to 9 inches apart, toes pointed out slightly.
2. Squat slowly until your armpits are over your knees.
3. *Caution:* you may initially have trouble with your balance. Be careful not to fall *backward*.
4. Allow your back to relax, with your head hanging in a relaxed position.
5. Sway slowly from side to side. Next sway slowly forward and backward in a similar manner, then in a circular fashion clockwise and counterclockwise.
6. Relax into the stretch for 30 seconds.
7. Repeat for a 45-second stretch.
8. Repeat for a 60-second stretch.

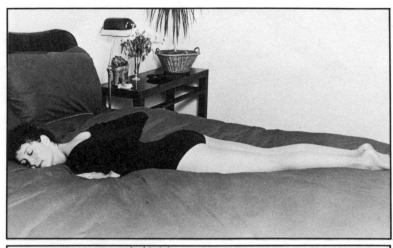

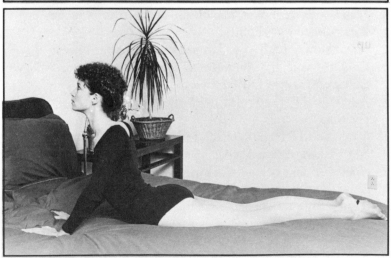

EXERCISE 12: McKenzie Press Up

1. Lie on your stomach and place your hands on the surface on which you are lying as you would for a conventional push-up.
2. Press your shoulders and upper body away from the surface, leaving your pelvis and hips on the surface.
3. Hold and relax in this up position for 5 seconds. Repeat ten times.

Note: As you begin this exercise, come only part way up until you feel confident and comfortable enough to come all the way up.

Note:

Sections of this book are condensed from Dr. Mulry's *Tension Management and Relaxation*, which is produced by the C. V. Mosby Company and consists of a complete Tension Management manual, Personal Concerns Inventory, and four half-hour tapes to aid Relaxation Therapy. The tapes are entitled "Gentle Rainfall," "An Evening With Nature," "Sounds of the Sea," and "A Quiet Place." To order them, call American Network Services at (714) 544-1398.